Economic Effects of Health Reform

C. Eugene Steuerle

The AEI Press

Publisher for the American Enterprise Institute

WASHINGTON, D.C.

1994

To order call toll free 1-800-462-6420 or 1-717-794-3800. For all other inquiries please contact the AEI Press, 1150 Seventeenth Street, N.W., Washington, D.C. 20036 or call 1-800-862-5801.

ISBN 0-8447-7019-1

THE AEI PRESS
Publisher for the American Enterprise Institute
1150 17th Street, N.W., Washington, D.C. 20036

ISBN 978-0-8447-7019-2

Contents

The health care market in the United States, and the government's role in that market, are already so large that even moderate changes in health care reform can have significant effects on the economy. Occupying more than one-seventh of the gross domestic product today, health care involves an average expenditure of about $9,500 per household. Taxpayers cover about half of all costs through federal, state, and local expenditures and tax subsidies—more, by the way, than is spent by taxpayers in many countries with national health insurance.

To reconfigure the government's role in that market in a way that can best improve total economic well-being is not an easy task. In this essay, I will concentrate on the potential effects of health care reform on five areas of the economy: (1) the federal budget; (2) the labor market; (3) the distribution of income; (4) innovation; and (5) the administration of health care. Each of these issues arises in conjunction with the administration's health care plan, and many also arise in the alternatives that lie before the Congress.

The Effects of Health Care Reform on the Federal Budget

Estimating Changes in Health Care Costs. Designing health care reform proposals involves an extraordinary amount of data analysis and research. Despite disputes over the cost of reform, the budget analysts making these calculations operate under a strong code of ethics. The numbers derived by civil service budget estimators are highly unlikely to be biased, but the reviewer of such numbers has to understand the limits of the budget estimators' authority, the assumptions under which their calculations are made, and the inability of existing data to answer crucial questions. My purpose here is to present the largest sources of uncertainty in the revenue and expenditure estimates accompanying health care reform. These issues cannot be determined easily by budget estimators, no matter how capable. These are also issues on which no consensus

Much of the material in this essay is based on articles that appeared previously in *Tax Notes, Policy Bites* (Urban Institute), *The American Enterprise* (American Enterprise Institute), and the author's testimony before the Ways and Means Committee.

is likely to emerge among policy makers, for the sources of potential disagreement often go to fundamental beliefs about how well government can or cannot operate.

Question one is, Are cost controls going to be effective? President Clinton's health care plan relies significantly on some form of cost constraint or control to limit future government health expenditures. In estimating the effect of its reform, the administration adopted a variety of goals for cost increases in various programs. Health costs in Medicare in a given year, for example, would be targeted under reform to grow only at inflation plus 3 percent. Private payments for insurance in another year would be targeted under reform to grow only at inflation plus 2 percent. And so on. The targeted growth in health care costs under reform would then be compared with a baseline projected cost increase absent reform. These projected costs absent reform are always assured to be higher than costs under reform.

Under these assumptions, budget estimators calculate how much costs would fall under reform budget targets relative to baseline health costs without reform for Medicare, Medicaid, and other federal programs, as well as the exclusion of employer-provided health insurance from individual taxation. A recent Lewin-VHI study[1] examined the administration's health plan and concluded that it might eventually reduce the deficit, although by less than the administration stated.[2] This conclusion, however, was made conditional on the presumed efficacy of the cost controls on premiums and prices—issues that were not examined in the study.

In truth, the debate over cost controls involves not one, but many, questions. Of what form is the cost control? In the administration's latest round, it suggests caps on premiums that could be paid, but other controls also have been considered. Can these be implemented administratively? Can they be maintained politically? Can they be calculated fairly across regions and in different time periods? What economic pressures do they put on the health system, and are those pressures containable? What are the associated efficiency costs in the economy? How will cost controls on private-sector behavior translate into cost saving in government programs? How do particular cost controls relate to goals for cost saving? Note that the budget estimator is not responsible for answering most of these questions. Regardless of personal views on the wisdom of different types of controls, the budget estimator is required to assume that they are put into the law and will remain there. A budget estimate is made on the assumption of the law's passing, as intended by its authors, and remaining permanently. Efficiency costs and political sustainability do not enter into the calculation.

A more difficult task faced by the budget estimator is to conclude whether the proposed law change can achieve its targets. The enforcement mechanisms, for example, must be administratively feasible. If there are easy ways to dodge federal proscriptions, then the budget estimator will not give those proscriptions much weight and the cost saving may not materialize. This is a difficult area, and budget estimators are often reluctant to make their numbers bounce around with various administrative designs.

Question two is, How much will a change in market incentives lead to a restructuring of the health marketplace? Almost all health care proposals, including that of the president, attempt to change incentives within the medical marketplace. The creation of a standard plan or plans, for instance, will cause individuals to be much more price-conscious when choosing their health insurance. In a like manner, individuals might choose insurance policies differently if they are allowed as employees to pocket any saving generated from choosing a lower-cost plan. Note that the more powerful these effects are, the less important the need will be for cost controls.

Question three is, How much will the demand for health care change as a result of the new law? In the Lewin-VHI study, currently uninsured individuals would increase their health spending by 60 percent under national health care reform. In addition, those who are currently insured would often benefit from better policies—thus expanding their own demand for health insurance. Under the administration's plan, however, all of the expanded demand might have to be met under the health premium caps. This would shift rather than increase health costs by constraining the supply of funds to meet all of the increased demand.

Demand also increases because of new benefits, such as drugs and long-term care under Medicaid. New benefits are sometimes limited by specifying a fixed amount of money to be turned over to the states, hence making the estimate independent of demand. Note again that political sustainability is not part of the estimate. Question four is, How much will the supply of health care change? Very little analysis has been given to this issue. Some speculation has been made about a possibly excessive supply of medical specialists in the future. This type of analysis, however, simply takes past trends, projects them into the future, and then tries to determine how new rules, say on medical schools or on payments to providers, will affect supply. Some other research has focused on the ability of physicians to increase volume when prices are cut. Changing the rules of the medical marketplace, however, will have an effect on such health institutions as medical schools, medical research organizations, and health insurance companies that is far greater than anything examined before. Innovative practices and procedures may contract or expand as a result of malpractice reform, cost controls, and other efforts. As suppliers change in quantity and quality, so also will the quantity and quality of health care provided.

Question five is, How much will employment change? Employment will likely decline under almost all health care reform proposals. An employer mandate effectively raises the minimum wage and raises the price of hiring such workers. More important, the availability of health insurance at only a small cost when income is low will lead to an increase in early retirement and longer spells of employment search. Suppose that employment falls by 1 million. This implies lower earnings of $35 billion if we assume lower-than-average productivity for the workers involved. This in turn translates to a loss of government receipts of about $10 billion at a combined effective tax rate on this income of a little less than 30 percent. In addition, as earnings fall, the cost of any health subsidy based on earnings or income will increase. The size of the employment shift, therefore, can have a significant effect on the budget. If the economy enters another recession, employment will fall below current estimates. This will further raise the cost of subsidies based on employment, earnings, and income. In addition, if health care reform increases employment search time, the full effect may not be felt until a recession occurs.

Question six asks, What is the time period over which these changes occur? Suppose we were able to know the long term employment effect of health care reform. How long will it take to get to the long-term? Estimators will assume some time lag, especially where behavior is changing. Little information is available, however, regarding the length of those prospective time lags.

Question seven is, What will happen to government health care costs under current law? To measure the effect of health care reform on the budget, one must know what will happen without reform. This requires a complete understanding of what is occurring in the medical marketplace today. This calculation is in many ways more difficult than the one estimating the change in the law. The estimate of the change, however, is greatly dependent on the baseline. If the baseline is too low (or high), for example, then estimated gains attributed to effective cost controls will be too high (or low).

None of these questions is easily resolved with existing data and models. In the end, policy makers will have to make decisions based on how well they expect particular policies are to perform in the economy as a whole, not on revenue and expenditure estimates that are inevitably uncertain.

Estimating Baseline or Current Law Health Costs. Many of the health proposals now before Congress start with the presumption that without reform the nation's health bill will rise from about one-seventh to one-sixth of economic output within a span of five years. From this presumption, most of the proposals, including the president's, conclude that to pay for reform, at least over those first five years, the nation must raise its health bill by a similar amount. I take issue with allowing this framework to guide health care reform.

Despite past growth in health care costs, such a massive shift would still be unprecedented, especially in its depressing effect on the nonhealth sectors of the economy. If the presumption is wrong, moreover, policy makers run the danger of converting a guess about future health spending into a minimum spending commitment. Under the Congressional Budget Office's 1993 projections, health spending under current law will rise from 14.6 percent of gross domestic product (GDP) in 1993 to 17.3 percent in 1998. After taking out inflation, real annual health expenditures would be about $320 billion higher in 1998 than in 1993. Federal, state, and local governments, meanwhile, cover about half these costs through direct expenditures and tax subsidies, so that by the end of the five-year period taxpayers would need to provide an additional $160 billion or so annually simply to pay for government health expenditures and subsidies.

These numbers are driven mainly by projections that growth rates of the recent past will continue. In each of four ten-year periods between 1948 and 1988, real health care spending per person, excluding growth caused by inflation and population increase, never grew more slowly than 3.9 percent or more rapidly than 5.7 percent (see table 1). Per person growth in real health spending has continued at the highest end of this scale (5.8 percent) over the past five years, so analysts in both the executive and the congressional branches project annual growth at 5.5 percent from 1988 to 1998.

Given plausible total growth, however, health care cannot grow this fast without having an effect on the growth rate of other goods and services provided in the economy. Projected growth for the nonhealth sectors can be approximated by subtracting projected health sector growth from total economic growth. All of a sudden constant real growth in health spending, at a rate significantly higher than total growth, is revealed to be not such a simple assumption after all.

Such growth is impossible to maintain unless the corresponding growth rate in nonhealth expenditures is nonconstant and declining. To take an example from business, it is one thing for IBM or General Motors or Exxon to grow faster than other firms while they are still small. But when they are giants, maintaining a higher-than-average growth rate implies absorption of huge increments of labor and other resources that would no longer be available to other firms. Based on current projections, health care would so dominate the economy that nonhealth expenditures per person would grow by an average of only 0.3 percent annually between 1988 and 1998. Put another way, increased health spending under current projections would capture 45 percent of GDP growth and 76 percent of growth in income per person.

This result is not impossible. Total real growth in the economy between 1988 and 1993 was so modest that per person spending on nonhealth expenditures went down. The decade-long projection of only 0.3 percent increase in per person nonhealth expenditures is composed of a recession-induced annual decline of -0.5 percent between 1988 and 1993,

TABLE 1
REAL SPENDING ON HEALTH CARE AND EVERYTHING ELSE IN THE UNITED STATES, 1948–1998
(constant 1993 dollars)

	Annual per Capita Growth in Spending (%)		Dollar Increase per Capita		Increase in Health Spending and GDP (%)	
	Health	Other	Health	Other	Total	Per Capita
1948–58	3.9	1.6	210	1,800	8	10
1958–68	5.7	2.8	490	3,910	9	11
1968–78	4.6	1.5	650	2,630	15	20
1978–88	4.0	1.2	870	2,370	20	27
1988–98	5.5	0.3	1,900	600	45	76

SOURCES: Historical data from Department of Health and Human Services and Bureau of Economic Analysis. Projections reflect 1993 Congressional Budget Office assumptions. Nonhealth expenditures are approximated as gross domestic product (GDP) less health expenditures. Calculations for 1988–1998 would be about identical under Clinton administration estimates for their own health reform package.

and a recovery rate of only 1.0 percent between 1993 and 1998. This can be contrasted with a recession-induced decline of -0.4 percent between 1978 and 1983, and a recovery rate of 2.8 percent between 1983 and 1988. The implications of such a trend are disquieting. Barring substantial and unexpected growth in the economy, the nonhealth sectors could be committed to a decade-long growth rate among the lowest in U.S. history, except for that during the Great Depression. Bringing down these health costs is one reason why health care reform is so high on the policy agenda. To minimize political damage, though, many health care reform proposals for the first five years are aimed at reallocation of the health dollar scheduled to be spent under the baseline, rather than at reduction.

The baseline numbers themselves, however, are only a guess, even if an educated one. Suppose the projection is wrong and that, absent reform, demand pressures would force faster expansion within the non-health sectors and lower health spending growth. The commitment to spending the baseline, represented in many of the health care reform proposals now on the table, could prevent the savings from such a slowdown from being reallocated to nonhealth purposes. By adhering to a baseline estimated now, health care reform runs the danger of converting a guess as to future spending into a commitment to make that amount of health spending *a minimum*. The potential losers include not simply the nonhealth sectors, but also those who would benefit from other government efforts related to education, training, youth development programs, and crime prevention. Of course, we should make headway on eliminating distortions in the health care market and expanding coverage for the uninsured. As a purely budgetary matter, however, a five-year government commitment to increase real spending on health by hundreds of billions of dollars must inevitably inhibit all other government actions. This, indeed, could easily be the principal economic effect of health policy over the next few years.

The Effects of Health Care Reform on the Labor Market

One of the most difficult issues in health care reform is the reaction of the many affected parties: workers, insurers, health care providers, and individual demanders of health care. Depending on their behavioral response to new potential incentives, costs could vary widely. The first part of any economic analysis is the assumption that individuals act in their own interest. They will try to minimize taxes and to maximize the benefits they receive from any government program. If tax rates are too high, individuals may choose not to work and may turn to alternative activities, such as leisure or retirement.

Although much concern has been expressed with respect to changes in the demand for health care as insurance and access are expanded, of equal importance is the extent to which employment rates would fall. A

7

decrease in employment reduces national production and income, while taxes collected on that income would fall and budget deficits would rise. Several aspects of the president's plan are relevant here.

Low-Income Workers. First, at very low wage levels the employer mandate in the president's plan has the same effects as tax on hiring or maintaining workers. At higher levels of wages, most of an employer mandate can eventually be passed on to employees through lower cash wages and smaller raises in wages over time. At minimum wage levels, however, the administration plan would require a typical employer to contribute an additional 7.9 percent of wages to purchase health insurance. Thus, the mandate operates in some ways like an increase in the minimum wage. If the worker's value of production is just at the minimum wage, then hiring or maintaining that worker can be done only at a loss.

There is much debate among economists about the effect of minimum wage changes on employment. In general, most believe that minimum wage effects are most pronounced for teenagers and some secondary workers, in part because most primary workers earn more than the minimum wage. Certainly an increase in the minimum wage has a modest effect on the level of wage at which employers can hire and test workers on their abilities—even if successful workers are likely to move up to higher wage levels. The administration would offset some of this by exempting dependent teenagers from any mandate.

Among many welfare recipients, the net effect of health care reform on work effort is probably positive. Many of these individuals are eligible for Medicaid payments under current law. When they do go to work, though, they often lose those benefits, especially after a transition period. In effect, the loss of Medicaid benefits operates much like a tax of up to several thousand dollars. With health care reform, a person moving to a job paying, say, $10,000 a year would pay no more than $1,000 to buy insurance that could be worth several thousand dollars. The effective "tax" generated by moving from welfare to work, therefore, would be reduced, and work would be made more attractive.

Congress is now considering the expansion of coverage under an approach that would eliminate benefits more quickly as income rose. When health benefits are phased out in this manner, as they were in a plan proposed by the Bush administration, the effective tax rates from direct taxes, from the phasing out of benefits, and from minimal costs of working create the Medicaid dilemma—tax rates of close to 100 percent over a significant portion of the income range. Because health care reform would no longer apply to particular categories of individuals, moreover, this type of approach effectively puts the entire population into a welfare-like tax structure during periods of low-to-moderate earnings. Marriage penalties deriving from this type of structure are also quite severe, often amounting to several thousand dollars per couple.

The employment effect on low-wage workers is also limited significantly by the special subsidy provided to employers with concentrations
of low-income workers. If a small company's payroll is less than $12,000
per worker, for instance, the employer cost for hiring an additional
low-wage worker could not exceed 3.5 percent (rather than, say, 7.9 percent), and the employee's share would be correspondingly less. This cuts
the equivalent increase in the minimum wage by more than half.

This sword, however, is two-edged. The proposed subsidies for
small employers are expressed as a cap on the percentage of payroll that
must be paid for health care. The government must spend a significant
amount of money to cover each subsidy. These subsidies, moreover, create
incentives for low-wage employees, including many who are well above
minimum wage, to migrate to the subsidized sector of the health care market. Larger firms and those with above-average wages would contract out
work required by low-income individuals to other firms. These shifts over
time would raise the total costs of the subsidies significantly.

Two-Income Households. Still another group likely to reduce its labor
supply is composed of households with more than one job. The economics
literature finds secondary workers in households more sensitive than
other groups to taxes and subsidies. Under the administration plan,
two-earner couples would be required to pay twice for their health insurance, as each employer would contribute regardless of coverage elsewhere
in the family. Many individuals considering working more than one job
also face a large increase in tax burden with no increase in benefits.

Retired Workers and the Elderly. Today's rising health costs occur in a
world where the numbers of new elderly are relatively small, not large.
When the baby boom generation begins to retire early next century, however, both health and retirement costs will rise dramatically. Among the
likely requirements for meeting those not-too-distant problems are grad-
ual increases in a retirement age, or constraints on the number of years of
public support for retirement—already being provided for an average of
almost two decades.

One of the principal employment effects of the administration plan,
however, comes from the voluntarily reduced labor supply of workers
themselves. The design of this plan, as well as other alternatives on both
sides of the aisle in Congress, provides that many nonworking individuals would have to pay only a moderate share of their unearned income to
cover the cost of insurance. Someone who retires early from the work
force, therefore, would often pay only a small amount—in many cases, a
few hundred dollars—for health insurance. A working person, however,
would pay directly or indirectly either about 10 percent of wages or the
cost of the plan. The cost of work relative to early retirement, therefore,
would rise significantly.

In effect, health care reform would provide a significant subsidy for earlier retirement at a time when the nation needs to be moving in the opposite direction. For those considering early retirement from the work force, the proposal provides a substantial subsidy for that retirement. Older individuals, whether they retire or not, would also be subsidized by the simple community-rating requirement in the administration plan. Under this requirement, the same price would be charged for all insurance, with exceptions for regions and size of household. Since individuals in their fifties have health insurance costs significantly higher than those of younger individuals, the requirement that the same price be charged to all age groups raises costs, especially for younger individuals, who on average are poorer than the middle-age and near-elderly persons they will subsidize.

The labor supply effects discussed so far focus on those who will spend longer times in job searches, those who decide to retire from the labor force, and those who avoid second jobs in the same household. In truth, some labor supply response might be expected from other parts of the labor force. For many individuals, the plan acts both like an increase in income from the government and like an increase in tax rates of about ten percentage points. The income from the government (in the form of guaranteed health insurance) is available even if the individual's own earnings are zero, while the tax is assessed either on earned income or unearned income. Both the income and the tax effects create incentives for reduced work effort.

These labor responses are difficult for any administration to discuss. Politics does not support such statements as, "Our bill would reduce employment by only...." In truth, however, almost all forms of increased social insurance involve changes in incentives. President Bush's health plan, for instance, also contained some significant work disincentives. The difficulty this time is that even if labor responses turn out to be modest per dollar of mandate or expenditure involved, the magnitude of the proposed changes is so large that the employment effects cannot easily be ignored.

The Potential Segregation of Workers by Economic Class. A number of difficulties are created by trying to design health care reform around mandates and subsidies on employers. The design of an employer subsidy in President Clinton's plan, for instance, leads to the *economic segregation* of workers, with the rich and poor workers becoming increasingly separated by the type of employer. This type of employer subsidy would be to health policy what old-time public housing was to housing policy in its effect on economic segregation.

This economic segregation, again, is an unintended consequence of policy design. It derives from the attempt to subsidize the employers of low-income workers rather than the low-income workers themselves.

Thus, the administration would set caps or maximum figures on the amount of expense that employers have to pay for health insurance, with even lower caps on small businesses whose employees have lower-than-average wages. These employer-based caps as a percentage of payroll effectively create incentives for low-wage employees, including many who are well above minimum wage are married to high-income spouses, to migrate to the subsidized sector of the health care market. Larger employers and employers paying above-average wages—that is, those employers who have less access to subsidies for their own low-wage employees—will contract out, or "outsource" work required by low-wage individuals.

Although the administration states that it will try to set legal limits on such outsourcing, no one believes these limits will be enforceable. Even if they are enforceable at first, labor markets have alternative ways of reorganizing to minimize cost. A firm that cannot outsource work already done by existing employees, for instance, will find that it becomes less competitive than a new firm that never hires those low-income employees in the first place. The latter, lower-cost firm will eventually dominate the market.

High-wage workers, meanwhile, would be induced to move toward firms that do not benefit from the subsidies for low-wage workers. Because of the design of the employer subsidy, the health costs of hiring high-wage workers would often be higher on average in the subsidized firms. This is merely the other side of the outsourcing problem.

Some examples clarify this problem. For simplicity, let us divide employers into three groups. Group A is composed of those employers (and employees) who do not benefit from the cap on health costs as a per-centage of average wages paid. They will be made to pay the full cost of the health plan. Assume that the employer-related assessment of a family policy for each employee is $2,500 in the year in question—a cost that is low relative to projected costs in later years of the proposal. Added to this will be an employee share that does not vary by type of employer, of about $870. The total cost of the policy will then be $3,370.

Group B is composed of those employers who face a maximum tax rate of 7.9 percent of payroll. Added to this again will be an employee cost of $870.

Group C involves those small employers who are eligible for even greater subsidies. Let us simplify matters and take only the case of those employers who face a maximum tax rate of 3.5 percent of payroll, sup-plemented by the usual $870 paid by the employee. We ignore possible separate subsidies to low-income individuals, which are available equal-ly no matter where they work, and which do not affect the differences in total cost.

Now ask the question, What does it cost to purchase insurance for an additional employee in each of these groups? If we ignore cases where

11

one additional employee forces the employer from one subsidized group to another, the answer is the following:

- insurance cost paid by an employer for an employee earning $10,000 a year:
  $3,370 in Group A — cost of insurance
  $1,660 in Group B — normal employer cap as percentage of payroll
  $1,220 in Group C — lowest cap for small business

- total private insurance cost of an employee earning $100,000 a year:
  $3,370 in Group A — cost of insurance
  $8,770 in Group B — large employer cap as a percentage of payroll
  $4,370 in Group C — lowest cap for small business

The last example—$4,370 for the $100,000 employee in Group C—would in most cases understate the additional cost of insurance for hiring this employee. The $100,000 salary likely would move the firm up into a lower subsidized rate for all employees—thus creating a very large increase in costs.

Powerful incentives, therefore, drive the $100,000 worker toward plans that are capped at the cost of insurance, and the $10,000-a-year worker toward plans with caps as a percentage of payroll. The government would effectively differentiate among individuals based simply on the type of employer for whom they worked—not the amount of their wages. Not only does this violate the notion of equal justice under the law, but it economically segregates the work force—an important social consequence.

This migration, by the way, will feed back into the system to increase the cost of subsidies. As workers and firms reorganize themselves to maximize the value of the government subsidy, they will pay less directly, and government's share of total cost will rise.

In many ways, this design is reminiscent of many public housing projects of the past. Instead of giving a subsidy more directly on the basis of individual need, the subsidy is passed through one or several qualified intermediaries. Individuals respond by working or living not where they wish, or where they would be most productive, but rather where subsidies are greatest. Is such economic segregation of the labor market really a goal of health care reform?

The Effects of Health Care Reform on Income Distribution

Budget and tax policy making in Washington are often driven by two sets of numbers: (1) the effect of a proposed policy change on expenditures, taxes, and the deficit; and (2) the distribution of the change among individuals. The health care reform debate so far has focused its attention on the former. Tables on the redistribution of net income caused by health care reform have not yet been released, either by the administration or by congressional agencies such as the Joint Tax Committee or the Congressional Budget Office.

Many advocates of health care reform believe they will achieve a substantial redistribution of income toward the poor and the near-poor. Economic analysis, however, shows that the details of program design often yield unintended consequences. Taxes, mandates, and subsidies are often paid by persons other than those on whom they are assessed. According to Urban Institute research by Sheila Zedlewsky, John Holahan, Linda Blumberg, and Colin Winterbottom, a number of national health care reform proposals—especially those involving mandates on employers—involve only a modest amount of redistribution to the poor and near-poor. While health care reform would redistribute hundreds of billions of dollars and would force payments to be made by different sources and through different intermediaries, the gain for the poor might still be only a few billion dollars. Modest welfare reform, in fact, would achieve more redistribution than many health care reform proposals.

To understand these results, health care reform must be divided into its many components. The combination of these pieces—some regressive, some progressive—leads to the total changes in redistribution. Here are a few important possible changes and how they might affect redistribution.

Employer Mandates. A mandate on employers to provide health insurance, it turns out, is often regressive. Economists believe that an employer mandate is eventually financed out of lower cash wages and that most employees pay individually for the cost of their own insurance. Hence, an employer mandate to buy health insurance at a cost of $3,000 will lower the employee's cash wages by $3,000 and raise pay in the form of employee benefits by an equal amount.

For those already buying insurance, the mandate may make little difference in either cash wages or employee benefits. A large portion of those who do not buy insurance, however, are concentrated among workers with low or moderate pay. Some of these have access to charitable care and some to Medicaid. When large health bills become due, these individuals often cannot pay; others provide subsidies indirectly by paying additional amounts on their own hospital and doctor bills. In effect, other members of society provide partial insurance, however inadequate, to those without insurance. Suppose this partial insurance on average is worth $1,000. When the employee is forced to forgo $3,000 in wages to receive a $3,000 health insurance policy, the net gain in insurance is only $2,000. Net income falls by the $1,000.

Another complication is caused by valuation. The employee may not value a $3,000 insurance policy at $3,000, regardless of whether or not other care is available. At low-income levels, food, clothing, and other necessities may take a higher priority in the budget. Indeed, health insurance is likely to be a good that rises in value and demand as income increases. This aspect of health care reform is not usually modeled.

Community Rating. Community rating has both progressive and regressive components, depending on how it is designed. The requirement to cover all people at the same price, no matter what their health condition, would transfer income from the healthy to the nonhealthy. The unhealthy tend to be worse off in both health and income, since they often have less capability for work. Hence, this part of the transfer is progressive. If community rating requires that the same price be charged to someone aged fifty-five as to someone aged twenty-five, however, community rating contains a regressive component. Why? Those who are older have higher health insurance costs, so they would receive net transfers. They also have higher incomes on average than those who are younger; hence this component of community rating requires transfers from poorer to richer.

Tobacco Taxes. The explicit tax structure also affects progressivity. Tobacco taxes, for instance, are regressive in nature.

Individual Subsidies. Subsidies are usually highly progressive. Even an equal-size grant per person or per household evens out the distribution of income. If the subsidy is phased out as income increases, the progressivity is even higher.

Employer Subsidies. To the extent that employer subsidies are concentrated on employers with lower-income employees, they will be progressive. Design, however, is crucial to ensure that the incidence of the grant is really with the employee, not the owners of the firm. In President Clinton's plan, some low-income employees in small firms would be helped and some in large firms would not be helped. Some higher-income individuals in small firms would also be helped, at least initially. A crucial issue is how long it takes for low-income employees to migrate toward firms where subsidies are greatest.

Behavioral Responses. Reform changes incentives. Individuals often change their patterns of work, for instance, to get the maximum benefit from the government. Under a number of plans offered by both Democrats and Republicans, subsidies would be based on current income. Therefore, many of those who retire early would substantially increase the amount of health insurance paid for by the government, and would reduce the amount for which they have to pay. The progressivity of the transfer will be calculated as much lower if individuals are counted on the basis of their original income. If distribution is shown on the basis of income after early retirement, however, the subsidy will appear more progressive.

Incentives and Controls. Suppose that new incentives or cost controls are successful in lowering the cost of health care. If cost is reduced, then either quantity of health care is reduced or the prices paid to providers are reduced. If prices are reduced, providers will likely provide less health care, and the health field will attract less qualified doctors and nurses.

No one likely will attempt to model the net effect of these changes, yet incentives and controls could drive the distributional outcome as much as any other factor. Much depends on whether the market is made more efficient. Even then, the changes at times could be regressive regardless of whether there is a net gain for society. Someone at zero income, for example, with comprehensive health insurance is almost bound to receive less health care if payments to providers are lowered.

Health care reform could easily involve the transfer of tens of billions of dollars of resources among individuals in society. Here are some of the possible winners and losers.

Those with and without existing health problems. Almost all proposals would attempt to guarantee the availability of health insurance to those who are sick. No longer could individuals be dropped from coverage, or even denied new coverage once they became sick. This is perhaps the principal concern of the middle class. The gain would be shared both by the sick and by all those who want, but cannot obtain, this protection against future health risks.

The issue of implementation is not a simple one. Either directly or indirectly, it will probably require a movement toward plans with more standard rates that apply across households. Pure community rating is an extension of this idea so that one insurance rate applies to everyone, except perhaps for adjustments for family size and geographical area.

Suppose at a minimum that reform limits adjustments in premiums for individual differences in health conditions. Those who come into the system with high health costs will then need to be subsidized by others. Perhaps a health alliance will offer some standard set of plans at a constant cost to everyone in the community. Perhaps insurance plans including employers who currently self-insure, will be required to accept and subsidize some portion of high-risk individuals who are not initially in their plan. Perhaps other insurance plans will be "taxed" to pay for a high-risk insurance pool. However the issue is worked out, it will require that someone pay for the transfers to cover the costs of those with extraordinary health needs. Of course, much of this already occurs, although inefficiently, in the current health system.

Those who purchase health insurance and those who do not. Many of those who currently avoid purchasing health insurance will no longer be able to do so under most health care reform plans. By not buying health insurance, they often fall back on charity care or public assistance when times go bad. Under reform, those currently uninsured would be required to buy insurance either directly or through an employer. Even modest plans, such as that sponsored by Senator Don Nickles and other members of the Senate, would assess a penalty for failing to buy health insurance.

Whether those who currently purchase insurance will be winners is another issue. Even though some of those currently without insurance would be forced to pay a greater share of costs, the number of those who are subsidized for their purchase of health insurance and the amount of health care subsidized are likely to rise.

Two-earner couples. Among the possible losers in health care reform would be two-earner couples. In the administration's plan, for instance, an employer will pay for insurance on behalf of all employees, regardless of whether they are covered under another household member's plan. Since the employee usually pays for these employer costs in lower wages, a two-earner couple could easily pay twice for health insurance.

In deriving its total plan structure, the administration recognized that these extra payments would be available to support the cost of insurance. That is, more payments for family policies would be made than there would be families. Therefore, the administration lowered the total price of a family policy—the price that would be paid by both employers and employees—to an amount below cost. As a consequence, the one-earner couples would receive a subsidy financed by the two-earner couples. This would often be true regardless of income level. Thus, two earners in a family with a combined income of $50,000 could contribute twice and pay much more than their share of insurance costs, while single earners in families with incomes of $100,000 could contribute once at an amount below cost.

Workers with more than one job. Workers with more than one job also could pay for health insurance more than once under a plan such as President Clinton's. Each employer would be required to pay on behalf of the employee, and likely wages would be reduced in every case. Just as in the case of the two-earner couple, the difficulty is caused by the presence of more than one job within the same household.

Elderly and teenage workers. Many teenagers work mainly for cash wages and obtain health insurance through their parents or guardians. Many elderly individuals work in jobs paying cash wages, because they receive health insurance in the form of Medicare. Once employers are no longer allowed to pay cash wages only but must also buy health insurance for all workers, both elderly and teen workers will face either reduced wages or fewer job opportunities. Here again, the problem is caused by the requirement to purchase health insurance twice.

The near-elderly and the young. If a plan adopts pure community rating, as suggested by the administration, then individuals of all ages will pay the same amount for health insurance. The cost of health insurance for those in their fifties, however, is several times greater than for those in their twenties. Since those who are older have greater health needs, at first this might be viewed as a transfer from those better off to those less well off. In fact, however, households of young adults generally have lower incomes than those of older adults. Indeed, statistics noting that children are now the poorest age group in the population are derived from household calculations that take into account the relatively lower wages of adults in their child-raising years. For many individuals in their fifties, the children have begun leaving the home, much of the mortgage on the house has been paid off, and peak lifetime earnings are being achieved.

Early retirees and workers. For nonworkers, the administration would charge a premium that is related to income. A Senate Republican bill would provide subsidies that also decline rapidly with income. In both cases, substantial encouragement for early retirement is given to someone willing to live on a moderate income. Perhaps the job is not enjoyable, there are enough assets and owner-occupied housing to live on, or later retirement income kicks in at a higher level. Once again, the younger part of the population would subsidize this increase in early retirement, either through higher premiums for its own insurance or through higher taxes paid to the government.

Firms with dangerous jobs. Another aspect of pure community rating, such as suggested in the president's plan, is that it would redistribute health costs from firms with relatively safe jobs to those with jobs where injuries are more prevalent. Thus, the cost of insurance for professional football teams or miners would be no different from that for any other employer, such as a retail store. Internal efforts to make jobs safer would be of no benefit to a firm when it purchased health insurance.

An important legal and economic tenet is that if firms are made to bear the cost of hazards they place on employees, they will be alert to ways minimizing those hazards. Absent such incentives, hazards in the workplace can be expected to increase. Professional sports teams, for instance, will pay less attention to developing rules that might cut back on injuries. Among other losers, therefore, are those who will suffer injuries that otherwise might have been avoided at a reasonable cost.

In sum, if progressivity is the goal of health care reform, many easier, cheaper, and less disruptive routes will get us there. The debate over health care is largely a debate over financing, the efficiency of the health care market, and the fairness of a system in which some pay and others do not. Based on standards of equity and efficiency, some of the winners and losers listed above seem reasonable and others quite unreasonable.

The Effects of Health Care Reform on Innovation

The long-term effect of health care reform on the economy depends more than anything else on what happens to innovation, both in the health and in the nonhealth sectors. Innovation itself is driven by the development of ideas and the ability of individuals to put those ideas to work—often against established interests.

Innovation within the nonhealth sectors of the economy can be restricted if the health cost increases discussed above are caused by artificial factors and perverse incentives. Innovation within the health care sector itself involves much more than research on new drugs or equipment. Among the many possibilities are the following:

- better preventive care, sometimes in exchange for less acute care
- the replacement of expensive providers with less expensive ones, especially where a standard set of practices or routines can be developed
- new forms of organization that are as evolutionary as preferred provider or health maintenance organizations were in their day
- new forms of insurance policies, perhaps with tighter price limits or better incentives for individuals to avoid hazards to their own health
- new practices of employer-employee bargaining that would give the employee more incentive to restrict amounts paid for health insurance
- a better information network within the health care sector, such as computerized shot records and the availability of written material to patients

But innovation is messy. It often creates inequities between those who initially benefit from the innovation and those who do not; it imposes costs on those who are the subjects of innovation that fails.

Health care twenty years from now will be drastically different from what we know today. Regulations applying well to today's market can easily become outdated obstacles to innovation in tomorrow's market. Given an existing supply of health providers and researchers, as well as a set of habitual practices by consumers, health care reform in its initial years will affect mainly the financing and distribution of health care, not the types of health goods and services provided. The long-term effect of reform on health, though, will be determined largely by whether new, cost-effective products and practices are encouraged or discouraged. In this regard, the existing health care market in the United States is innovative, in part because of its vast increase in funds. However, it has too few incentives for its innovation to be cost effective. In other innovative markets, for instance, the prices of existing goods and services often fall rapidly as new goods and services are made available. Most boards regulating health care are composed of today's providers and consumers—not tomorrow's. The new health care providers and the new firms of tomorrow are not even represented in these political processes.

Governments, too, must be able to innovate, as knowledge expands and new needs arise. The budget dilemmas of today, as well as complaints about stagnant policy making, arise from the precommitment of all of tomorrow's finances before tomorrow has arrived. The more that government policy for tomorrow gets determined today, the less able will government be to take advantage of innovative opportunities that arise tomorrow.

The Effects of Health Care Reform on the Administration of Health Care

Mixing Employer and Individual Mandates. Despite the attention given in the Clinton health plan to mandates that employers purchase health insurance for their employees, the proposal also contains an individual mandate that has been given very little attention. Any proposal to move toward more universal coverage, in fact, will almost inevitably contain such a mandate.

Regardless of merits, an employer mandate is insufficient to address the lack of health insurance throughout the population. Many individuals without insurance do not work. The administration, therefore, proposes a separate mandate and subsidy scheme to deal with them.

If an employer mandate is not backed by an individual mandate, the only other way to move toward universal coverage is to subsidize all nonworkers. The idea of subsidizing millionaires who decide not to work, however, is not appealing. Once it is decided that these millionaires must pay some portion of cost, the issue of an individual mandate is engaged and a whole series of decisions is required. What about those with slightly less than $1 million? What are the penalties or taxes on those who do not buy insurance under the mandate? If some workers are required to pay more than the cost of their insurance to subsidize others, should rich nonworkers also be required to contribute something extra?

A strong and convincing rationale lies behind a mandate requiring the purchase of insurance. The principal arguments are efficiency and equity. Most industrial societies provide some backup health insurance to all individuals who are in need of medical care but have not purchased their own health insurance. This backup insurance may take the form of

Medicaid or charitable care. Other individuals have purchased their own insurance so that, when bad times arrive, they have prepaid to cover their needs. Among those who fall back on government or charity, however, there are many who were equally capable of paying for some or all of their insurance. Those who buy insurance, therefore, often pay more than their share of total costs. The back-up insurance system, moreover, gives everyone some amount of incentive to avoid purchasing insurance.

Mandates for insurance coverage try to solve some of these problems. Automobile insurance is a good example. All drivers are required to buy this insurance. While the mandate is not perfect—reckless drivers still take more from the system than they pay—at least it avoids the problems created by uninsured motorists.

These equity and efficiency arguments for mandates, however, apply to individuals. Today we would not think of requiring employers to provide automobile insurance. The inequities between those who buy and those who do not buy automobile or health insurance are not based on size of firm or any other employer-related variable. Similarly, if one wants to subsidize low-income individuals to buy insurance, then the subsidy is best based on individual, not employer, characteristics.

Employer mandates and employer subsidies create new, needless sources of inequity and inefficiency. They would discourage work at minimum wage levels. They would subsidize some of the rich. They would give different amounts of subsidy to two individuals who are equal in all respects except for the type of firm in which they work.

There is almost no rationale other than political to favor an employer mandate over an individual mandate. Although almost all economists believe that employer mandates are paid by workers mainly in the form of lower wages, many voters are convinced that employer mandates somehow tax employers. By hiding costs the employees would pay, the employer mandate is believed to be more politically appealing.

Some advocates also argue that employer mandates rely more directly on an existing system of employer insurance. Even under an individual mandate, however, employers could be required to offer insurance—thus not only maintaining but actually strengthening their role.

When an employer mandate is meshed together with an individual mandate, as in the administration's plan, the problems are compounded. For one, the distinction between those subject to an employer mandate and those subject to an individual mandate is not easy to make. A system of combined mandates must be created for uninsured individuals who work only parttime. In the administration's proposal, the employer mandate would cover a share of insurance cost approximately proportional to the number of hours worked per week, divided by thirty hours. Then the individual would be responsible for two remaining components: (1) the same share of the employer mandate that would be required of full-time employees; and (2) the portion of total health insurance cost that was not covered through the employer mandate. Suppose that an employee worked fifteen hours per week, for example, and that the employer generally split the cost of insurance with workers on an eighty to twenty basis—80 percent for the employer and 20 percent for the employee. Then the employer would cover 80 percent of one-half of total cost, or 40 percent of the total. The employee would be required to pay for the remaining 60 percent—fifty percentage points deriving from the individual mandate and ten percentage points as the matching payment required under arrangements with the employer (that is, 20 percent of the one-half required under the employer mandate). Furthermore, the administration proposes separate schemes for subsidizing or capping employer payments and for subsidizing individuals separately for their own payments.

This scheme of mixing and matching employer and individual mandates and subsidies is not only confusing—it is not administrable. Among other reasons, there is no reliable system for measuring the hours worked by individuals, and the employer mandate is based on hours worked. In addition, the number of hours worked one week may be different from the number worked the next, so that the required size of the mandate and the subsidy would either vary constantly over time or depend on some estimate based on earlier data.

Nonfilers. Testifying before the Ways and Means Oversight Subcommittee on October 26, 1993, IRS Commissioner Margaret Richardson indicated that nonfilers pose one of the most significant problems facing tax administration today. Current estimates, she indicated, imply that approximately 10 million individuals and businesses have not filed returns they should have filed. Approximately 7 million of these are individuals, many of whom work independently (so-called independent contractors) or own their own businesses.

On the same day, the administration began the formal release and presentation of material related to its health care reform proposal. A package of "financing material" dated October 26, 1993, indicated ways in which individuals and employers would pay for health insurance or receive premium subsidies under health care reform. Employer shares of premiums would be based on the number of hours worked a week, on the size of the employer and the average wages paid, and on certain other factors. Individual premiums, in turn, would be determined by a variety of factors in different combinations, such as the number of hours worked in a week and the amount of nonwage income.

The two discussions, both coming from the same executive branch at the same time, were never related to each other. In health care reform, no detailed discussion was held of administrative issues related to premium collection. In the nonfiler testimony, no reference was made to similar problems that might be created in health care reform.

Let us take some of the examples from a package of "Scenarios under Reform" released by the administration. This package provided examples of payments required by or on behalf of a variety of individuals in hypothetical situations. James Huggins, a hypothetical farmer earning $25,000 a year, would pay $872 as an individual and $1,975 as his own "employer." The latter amount is capped at 7.9 percent of the $25,000 of income. Lee Harris, who delivers pizzas twenty hours a week, would pay $386 per year, while his employer would pay $1,033 a year. The government would cover the rest of the employer cost, since he has no nonwage income. Mary Worthheimer, however, does have a nonwage income of $60,000 a year from her husband's estate, while earning $6,000 a year at a shop. She, therefore, will pay $1,419 in premiums, while her employer will chip in $516. Or so we are told.

Now wait a second. Whatever happened to those 10 million nonfilers? What if James hides some of his income? Does Lee spend some of his time working in the neighborhood, and receive income from mowing lawns and shoveling snow? What if Mary buys tax exempt bonds whose interest is not reported to the government, and she simply does not file a tax return? The Internal Revenue Service already indicates that it has been less than fully successful at keeping track of these individuals and ensuring that they pay annual taxes to the Treasury. One major reason is that it is quite expensive to send auditors after individuals, and the pickup of a few hundred dollars in tax is often less than the cost of the enforcement effort. A related reason is that there is a great deal of noncompliance elsewhere, and those enforcement efforts, while often more productive, eat up what resources are available to the IRS. Existing collection problems concern a tax system that relies on annual income accounting.

Now let us add to this a health mandate-tax-accounting system. Would the IRS or some health premium collection agency increase significantly its efforts to go after the 10 million nonfilers, many of whom presumably would not file a health premium return, or whatever it would be called? In addition to the 10 million nonfilers, what would be done to pursue those who paid too little over the course of the year because the withholding scheme or estimated health premium (like an estimated tax) was too low?

This health mandate-tax-accounting scheme, as currently designed, would often be far more detailed and elaborate for the typical individual than is the individual income tax. One reason is that the health accounting system would rely partly on weekly or monthly accounting. After all, an employer paying the employer mandate and withholding the employee share of premiums in January cannot know what the employee's income will look like in December. Determination of the employee's share in January would be based on January circumstances of the worker, but for low-income or less-than-full-time workers it would have to be adjusted over the course of the year.

The new health care reform also relies partly on an annual accounting system. How else is it going to charge appropriate additional premiums to individuals with nonwage income, to allow for rebates to individuals with multiple jobs, or to adjust for portions of the year in which work is done parttime (and, hence, individuals must pay a greater share of cost)? In order to administer this new system, moreover, individuals and employers must coordinate information. The individual presumably must report the number of employers and hours worked at each place so as to ensure appropriate withholding at each place for his share of costs. If he changes the number of hours worked at different places each week, a new report should be filed. Meanwhile, different regions or alliances must coordinate information to keep track of individuals moving from one area to another in the same year and facing different premium rates.

Even if these rather complex accounting schemes were workable, they would inevitably add to the noncompliance problem. Complexity not only causes error; it provides an excuse to those who are noncompliant in the first place.

The new payment mechanisms would also rely heavily on "hours worked per week." Currently there are no universal reporting requirements for employers, employees, and self-employed individuals on hours worked per week. Since the new system would base certain payments on these hours worked, new enforcement mechanisms and rules would be required to determine whether hours worked were reported appropriately. There is no discussion of how or whether such enforcement is even possible.

In blunt truth, this proposed system of mandates and subsidies is not administrable as currently designed. If Congress or the administration is to succeed in enacting some form of health care reform, it had better learn how to take into account information readily available to it—in some cases, provided to the public at the same time by its different, uncoordinated hands.

Conclusion

Health care reform is most likely to succeed as an economic matter only if a building-block approach is used. Before we have an intense debate over the furniture for the penthouse, we have to pay attention to these building blocks. Each must be examined individually to determine its costs, its value when added to the structure as a whole, and its relationship to its surroundings. We have to choose explicitly how much to spend on public provision of health versus other public goods. We must examine each aspect of community rating to see exactly how it affects incentives toward better health and safer environments, and whether it transfers from the well-off to the less well-off, or viceversa. Finally, we must give a great deal of attention to the side effects of attempts to subsidize small employers and low-income persons, such as effects on retirement policy or on the economic segregation of the work force.

Notes

1. Lewin-VHI, Inc. "Health Care Reform by the Numbers: An Assessment of President Clinton's Health Security Act" (December 9, 1993).

2. See *Tax Notes*, December 20, 1993, p. 1,417.

About the Author

C. EUGENE STEUERLE is senior fellow at the Urban Institute and author of a weekly column, "Economic Perspective," for *Tax Notes*. At the Urban Institute, he has conducted extensive research on budget and tax policy, health care, social security, and welfare reform. Earlier in his career, he was appointed deputy assistant secretary for tax policy for the Department of Treasury. In that role he directed the Treasury study *Financing Health and Long-Term Care: A Report to the President and the Congress*. Dr. Steuerle also serves or has recently served as an adviser, consultant, or board member to the American Tax Policy Institute, the Ways and Means Committee of the U.S. House of Representatives, the International Monetary Fund, and he is the National Commission on Children. He is president of the National Economists Club Educational Foundation.

AEI Studies in Health Policy

Special Studies in Health Reform

Other AEI Books on Health Policy

www.ingramcontent.com/pod-product-compliance
Lightning Source LLC
Jackson TN
JSHW011944131224
75386JS00041B/1562